Love Like That

Weekly Readings for Your Yoga Class & Your Life

by:
Cathrine Goldstein

Drishti Press

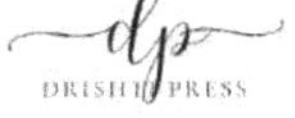

Copyright © 2023 Cathrine Goldstein All rights reserved

The characters and events portrayed in this book are fictitious. Any similarity to real persons, living or dead, is coincidental and not intended by the author.

No part of this book may be reproduced, or stored in a retrieval system, or transmitted in any form or by any means, electronic, mechanical, photocopying, recording, or otherwise, without express written permission of the publisher.

ISBN-13: 9798394694646

Cover design by: Drishti Press

Library of Congress Control Number: 2018675309

Printed in the United States of America

Website: www.MyDharmicJourney.com
@mydharmicjourney

Dedication:

This book is dedicated to all of my yoga students and teachers.

I thank you all for what you've taught me.

To all my unknowing muses—thank you.

Above all, thank you to Jay, Penelope, and Pickle

Please Note: Circumstances of stories have been changed to protect the privacy of individuals. The circumstances of my personal stories have not been altered.

Dear Yoga Teacher:

Hello! I am honored that you have decided to read, *Love Like That: Weekly Readings for Your Yoga Class & Your Life.*

This book is intended to help you as you theme your weekly classes.

Each reading is designed to be read in its entirety in a reasonable amount of time (for an average sixty minute drop-in class), or, you may choose to use only parts of the readings.

The italicized line or lines, either highlight the theme of the reading, or serve as a theme on their own.

And, if you do not feel like using the reading that week, I hope the theme will still inspire you in some way.

Finally, there are bonus poems in the back of the book. These can be used in conjunction with the readings— maybe at the end of class to tie up your theme—or, in place of a reading.

However you decide to use this book, I truly hope it helps you as you go forward with your important work. Yoga has the power to change the world in the most positive of ways.

Namaste,
Cathrine

Dear Reader:

Hello! I am so glad you have chosen to read, *Love Like That: Weekly Readings for Your Yoga Class & Your Life.*

This book is designed to offer you a weekly reading to contemplate as you go about your busy life. Maybe it will even offer a new way to look at things.

In yoga classes, we give themes for our students to consider as they practice. Our desire is that the theme may serve as an inspiration in their life off of the mat as well.

My hope is that this book serves as a similar guide for you.

Be well,
Cathrine

Table of Contents

Readings

Table of Contents

Poems

Success

Me

This Time Upon the Earth

Week One: **New Year, New Day**

Don't start this new year (or this new day, or this new month) by promising yourself that this will be your best ever.

Promising yourself that this new year will be the best year ever can make each moment of each day filled with too much pressure.

We compare this year to last, and we grow sad if things that we consider less-than-fabulous happen. And then, only months in, that "thing" happens, and we're ready to write off the entire year.

Rather than committing to an unrealistic idea that this has to be the best year ever, what if you go forward into this year (this day, or this month), simply experiencing it for what it is?

What if you make plans and work toward goals, but stop measuring and comparing this date to other years and experiences?

You were different then, you're different now, and you'll be different in years to come.

Yes, we all have years that stand out—the year we were married or had a child, the year we graduated or started a new job. Those years will always be special.

But it doesn't mean the others don't have merit.

In truth, I hope this year is the best year you've lived yet, and the worst of all to come.

But I've lived long enough to know that this year will probably be a year like other years—meaning, some days are going to be spectacular, and other days, less so.

But that's okay. That's life.

What really matters is that you are here and you are alive, and that makes this year pretty damned special just as it is.

So let's welcome the new year (day or month) without any undue pressure. Without comparing it or setting it up for failure. Without worrying that it has to be the best.

Let's look at this new year as a year to be brave, to open our hearts, and to lead with love, not fear.

Welcome New Year, with all your crazy ups and downs.

We are grateful to meet you.

Week Two: **Not Every Day is a Day to Create**

Not every day is a day to create.

Some days are to sit and listen, some are to walk in the woods, some are to read and be inspired, some are to remember to breathe deeply, some are to explore, and some are just to be.

Honor all your days.

Week Three: **Manifestation Miracles**

One rainy day, I was walking my dog when I looked down and caught a glimpse of my boot in a puddle. The oddest feeling came over me then, not quite déjà vu, but something similar. It was a powerful feeling of having manifested that very moment.

Often, when we think about manifestation, we think about the big things. We glue pictures of yachts and synonyms of "peace" to our vision boards, and we're very clear when we speak to the Universe, asking for help in manifesting our dream career.

But so often, we forget the small things we've had a hand in creating, like those millions of little miracles in our lives…those wishes we were granted.

As I stood there with my boots in the puddle, I remembered that at one time in my life, I had seen myself as an older woman, happy and content, walking my dog in the rain. And there it was. I had become the person I always imagined I would be. The person I wanted to be. *How lucky I am*, I thought.

Those small moments of manifestation miracles can sneak up on us. There's no fanfare, no announcement of their arrival. They are simply there. But if we're still and quiet, if we turn away from distraction and inward toward peace, we can recognize the miracle in the moments that we had a hand in designing, and that we're lucky enough to live.

Week Four: **People Need to Learn From You**

People need to learn from you. They need to know what you've been through and how you keep going. They need to know your life experiences, no matter how mundane they seem to you. They need to know what your dreams were as a child, and how you've evolved since then. They need to know how you've kept going for all this time despite the weight of the world crashing down on you. Despite love and loss. Despite life and death. They need to know that they too can plant a garden and feel better in the warm July sun, if only for a moment. They need to know that they can achieve their dreams at the age of ninety.

That time is not a barrier to hope. That there is a reason to keep going.

They need to learn from you that even though you lost the tournament and your dream job, even though someone you've loved has passed and you live in a place you never expected, even though your joints are stiff and that you've faced fear more times than you can count—

Even though. Even though.

They need to know that you have just kept going.

Week Five: **Go Your Own Way**

At one exceptionally challenging time in my life, most of the people in my immediate family were in talk therapy. Their therapy usually required my presence as well, which meant I was in therapy several times per week. That wasn't all, days were spent analyzing sessions, and before and after their meetings were heavy discussions and a great deal of unpacking. All of it was exhausting.

As an antidote for the round the clock stress I was feeling, I was also urged to see a therapist. Initially, I agreed that it could be useful. My plan was to unpack the weight I was carrying, so that I could continually hold space for others.

What I found instead was even more stress.

The very last thing I needed at that point in my life was more discussion. Although the topic of conversation shifted from them to me, it was still talking.

What I needed was to listen.

I needed to turn inward to a quiet place inside and hear what I had to say. I needed time to myself, and by myself.

So, I replaced weekly talk therapy sessions with another type of therapy: listening. As I walked in the woods on chilly winter mornings, I listened to the wind. As I sat beneath a tree in spring, I listened to the birds. When I strolled the neighborhood on late summer evenings, I listened to the cicadas. And in autumn, while I collected fallen pinecones beneath a tree, I listened to the rustle of leaves.

And finally, above all, I listened to myself.

Week Six: **There is a Power Greater Than You**

For a long time, I believed it was my job to fix everything for everyone I loved. It was experience, not Ego, that taught me if I didn't do it, then surely the problem would get worse. So, I accepted my given job and did the best I could, from the little things like driving family members to appointments and smoothing over hurt feelings, to the more serious issues of helping loved ones as they battled illnesses. And the more I did, the more that was piled onto me. Finally, one day, the weight of others' needs was so oppressive, I could no longer breathe. So I went to the woods, fell down beneath a tree, and surrendered. It was there, in that moment of surrender, that I felt calm, settled, and cared for. Something greater than me was supporting me and holding me up. Something greater than me was doing for me what I had been doing for others. Something greater than me told me to rest, and then urged me to go home with newfound hope.

Something greater than me was present.

You are not responsible for everything.
You don't need to do everything.
You cannot be everything to everyone.

You are not alone.
There is a power greater than you.

Week Seven: **Do What Feels Good**

Why do we dismiss the things that feel good to us and do more of what doesn't? When did we decide that to accomplish more, we had to be overworked and miserable? Why do we feel guilty about something as necessary as self-care?

Somewhere in your life, you may have been told—either directly or indirectly—that if you were enjoying yourself, it wasn't okay. Or, it was okay to enjoy for the moment, but not on a long-term basis. Eventually, you were told to stop whatever it was that you were enjoying, and get back to work. "All good things must come to an end," you may have been warned.

But it doesn't have to be so.

You can accomplish more when you're feeling good about what you're doing. Misery, and all its disciples—indigestion, ulcers, headaches, anxiety—together offer cues that something in your life is off track. Misery is not a badge to wear or a marker of excellence. "Powering through" doesn't make you a better person.

Do what feels good to you. Practice self-care without guilt or shame.

Doing more of what's making you miserable is counterintuitive. Your mind and body know what's right for you, so listen to them and let them lead.

We were meant to feel good in our bodies and minds, so stop forcing yourself into a tight, little box of misery.

Week Eight: **To Thine Own Self Be True**

You, and you alone, know what you truly need right now.

There was a time in my life when I was overwhelmed with stress and anxiety. In my personal world, people were battling varying mental illnesses, Alzheimer's was a part of our life, death and grief loomed—and all of it compounded at one time. Add in my own personal challenges, and most days, I simply wanted to run away.

But running was not an option.

The people I loved most saw the mountain of stress I was buried under, and offered their advice: "Rest," they suggested. "You need rest." Then they added chocolate and relaxation to the list, and summed it all up by saying I needed to do less for everyone, and more for me.

I appreciated the advice, but my heart and soul knew it wasn't quite right. They wanted something different.

We want to run away, they told me.

But running was not an option. Besides, I didn't really want to desert my responsibilities, I just wanted a break.

Then, I began noticing small things in my life that reminded me of a time a decade earlier when I was feeling my best physically, emotionally, and spiritually. There were signs my heart and soul picked up on: the name of a company who sponsored a road race I ran years ago, suddenly showed up in an online search. Thoughts of running with a baby stroller popped into my brain. My favorite running shoes, tucked deep in the back of the closet, made an appearance during a quick spring cleaning.

Then it hit me—the reason I was noticing these signs. What my heart and soul wanted me to know was that they wanted to *run*, not necessarily *run away*.

So I did. And once I started running again—even the shortest distances when I could find the time—my stress became more manageable, and I was able to be more present for my loved ones who needed me.

Shakespeare explained it best. *"This above all: to thine own self be true, And it must follow, as the night the day, Thou canst not then be false to any man."*

Do what you need to do. You know what that is. Look for the little clues, they're there. Thank the people in your life for their suggestions, but above all, follow your heart and soul and their infinite wisdom.

Week Nine: **Give the Younger Version of Yourself a Hug**

Facing our past selves can be difficult. As we grow, we have the luxury of creating the person we want to be. Often, it is not the person we once were.

But that doesn't mean the past you doesn't deserve love.

That past you did the best they could in that given situation. As the great Maya Angelou said, "Do the best you can until you know better. Then, when you know better, do better."

Don't leave the child, teen, or young adult you, behind. Don't leave them festering in their unhappiness. Go to them. Tell them you understand. Be the friend they never had. Tell them you understand why they made the choices they did, and show them how far you've come—together. Appreciate your past self. Without that past you, the you of today could not exist.

So take a deep breath and go to the you that you once were. Accept them exactly as they were, and then give that younger version of yourself a hug.

Week Ten: **You're a Bestseller**

When my first book became a bestseller, I thought there would be a seismic change in my existence. I was already happy with my life, but like most of us, I envisioned more. And, I was certain my book title on a certain list was the way to get there.

While there are some advantages to having a bestseller, the truth is, *nothing really changes*. In time, your book title leaves the list, and all you're left with is, well, you.

That's why it's you—and not a list—that will ultimately make you happy.

Happiness cannot come from an external place. Sure, a situation may feel good for the moment, but that's fleeting happiness, not true happiness. Happiness stemming from a bestseller list means giving power to external validation. In truth, the only validation that matters is the one that comes from you.

Every one of us is the author of our own story, so make sure the story you tell is truthful and authentic to you. It doesn't matter if anyone else likes it; you don't need their approval or their lists.

Embrace your story as the bestseller it already is.

Week Eleven: **Smart Does Not Equal Careful**

There may have been a time in your upbringing when you were told, "Make smart choices," or "Be smart."

Those statements may have started in earnest and with the best of intentions. When you were young, they may have been to remind you not to run into a busy street, and when you were older, they may have been said to warn you not to drink and drive, or to stay off drugs.

Sometimes, we begin to equate "being smart," with being careful. We're applauded every time we get an "A" in a subject we'll never use again, but we're reprimanded when we stay up 'til dawn to experience the beauty of a sunrise. We're told we're a "good kid" when we don't go to a wild concert with our friends, and "bad" when we do. We're "smart" when we do something society would approve of, and "stupid" when we follow our heart's desire.

But as we grow older and the moments and experiences begin to blend together, the times that we most often remember are those times when we rebelled. We probably don't remember doing our taxes (the smart thing to do), but we do remember staying up to see the sunrise, and the feeling of freedom we had when that band we snuck out to see all those years ago, played some song we've long since forgotten.

We think of being "smart" as being unadventurous and undaring, but nothing could be farther from the truth. Being "smart" means living your best life. Being "smart" does not mean lying on your deathbed regretting everything you might have done.

So be smart. Live in a way that is authentic to you. Explore, and try new things.

Being smart does not mean being careful. We're here to live our lives, to explore, and to dare.

Week Twelve: **Don't Be the Best**

There is so much pressure in the world today to be the best at everything. From our earliest days in school, we're taught to compete against each other. We have to get better grades, be captain of the wrestling team, get the lead in the play. If we don't, our life won't be… what, exactly?

That's the part they forget to tell us. What won't our lives be? Happy? Fulfilled? Joyful? Successful?

Truthfully, our lives have a better chance of being all of those wonderful things if we stop worrying about someone else and their track, and instead, focus on our own. And who decides who is the best, anyway? Is Maya Angelou a better writer than Toni Morrison, Virginia Woolf, or Harper Lee? Who decides?

And why does it matter?

To grow and develop in your life, try new things—things that your soul is aching to do. When you're old, will it be better to look back at your empty life and say, "Well, I never risked not being the best!" Of course not.

It's better to build a life rich in experiences, filled with a variety of things, some that you excel in, and others that simply bring you joy.

So go forward, try things, fall down and get up, get lousy reviews and stay up too late. Laugh it off. Stop comparing yourself to others, and above all, be the happiest you *possible. That's where true success lies.*

Week Thirteen: **Tough Love**

Here's a little tough love for you.

The person you're working so hard to prove wrong, the person who hurt you all of those years ago, probably doesn't remember that it happened. In fact, there's a chance they don't remember you at all.

What you are working so hard to create, the legacy you're leaving behind, won't mean much to future generations who are filled to capacity with their own cluttered thoughts, love affairs, and creations. They'll be focused on what's current. Their finger will be on their pulse—not yours. So stop worrying about what the world will think of you, because truthfully, most of them aren't thinking of you. In any way.

So write your damned novel, and stop worrying about what others will think. You won't make everyone happy no matter what you do. Wear purple socks, dye your hair green, study Lepidopterology, or whatever floats your boat. Get out of the office, or the lab, or your house. Take a walk in the sun, explore your local city, travel the world, learn new customs and languages.

Do whatever the hell you want, because the brutal truth is, *we only have this one go. Why would you live it for anyone but you?*

Week Fourteen: **Be Possessive of Your Time**

I once had a meditation teacher who turned an hourglass over at the start of every class. As far as I could tell, he didn't use it to judge the length of the session, he simply left the glass next to his mat and as the sand fell in a simple stream from top to bottom, he spoke, without any acknowledgment of the passage of time.

One day, I asked him why the hourglass was there when it was obvious he wasn't using it. "But I am using it," he told me. "I'm just not using it like you expect me to. For me, the hourglass is not a measure of time, but rather, *a remembrance of time and how precious it is*. The sooner we realize that this is all there is, the better off we are and the more possessive of our time we become."

Too many of us are trained to live "later." We push through work to get to drinks at happy hour, then we survive the work week, holding on for the weekend. For some reason, we willingly throw away huge chunks of the only finite, nonreplaceable thing in our life—time.

Be possessive of your time. While it's true that work cannot be avoided, clocking hours of misery doesn't make you worthier of enjoyment later. There is no later. There is only now.

Now is the time to live. Life is comprised of millions of moments, marked by memorable events that occur on an invisible timeline. But a minute is a minute of your finite life. No matter how it's spent. And you are only gifted so many minutes.

So, be possessive of your time, because every minute counts.

Week Fifteen: **Treat Yourself with Kindness and Compassion**

There are days that we're simply not feeling one hundred percent ourselves. Nothing is particularly wrong or bad, but we feel withdrawn, and we just don't want to put ourselves out there.

That's okay.

On those days, our minds and bodies are telling us they need some protection—they need to be treated with kindness and compassion. They need a little less attention from the world, and more attention from us.

I call these days our "Turtle Days." Days when we need the safety of our own shells.

We don't always need to power through, push through, or fight through. There are days we just need to pull back and be.

Some days, you may not have the luxury of a day off or even a few hours to recharge, so on those days, consider protecting your energy in a million little ways. Take a cup of tea to your meeting, participate by observing and listening not creating and doing, sit toward the back of the room rather than front and center, don't answer the question, wear your comfiest cardigan—the one that drapes around you—twice, try a Yin or Restorative Yoga class, eat a sweet pastry or three, start your day with a quiet meditation, end your day under a warm blanket watching

reruns of *Law & Order SVU*, and above all, hug those you
love and who love you.

It's okay to disappear into your shell for a day (or even
longer) if that's what you need. Honor what you're feeling.

Week Sixteen: **You Can't Rush the Seasons of Your Life**

We were fortunate to have an early spring this year. While areas of the world were digging out from late-winter snow storms, the Dogwoods in our backyard were blooming great white puffs of flowers. How lucky, we all agreed.

Suddenly, the cold came back, and the flowers that had made an impressive early start, now withered and died, falling before they were fully bloomed. All that was left behind were bare branches and a blanket of snowy white blooms beneath the tree. We got our snow after all, we all decided.

But then, when the calendar announced that spring had arrived, the trees were unseasonably bare.

Seasons cannot be rushed, and life is really no different.

We all want an early spring, but there is a reason bread rises before its baked, and seeds become seedlings before they can bloom. There is a natural evolution in our world that exists inside each and every one of us. Trust it.

Take time in your life. Breathe deeply and understand that all things need time to form.

When we rush through the seasons of our lives, we also stop blossoming before we've reached our true potential. Our life was designed to experience all moments of all of its seasons—from the coldest winter to the brightest summer days. All of it, together, support the life we live.

That is how we build. That is how we flower. That is how we bloom.

Week Seventeen: **Take Some Time to Bask in Who You Are**

One day, I was walking down lower Broadway and noticed a young woman on the street. She was sitting behind a table that was covered with her art—tiny paintings for sale. She was wearing paint splotched overalls, and her skin was speckled with matching paint dots. She was leaning back in a folding chair with her eyes closed; a rare sight in New York City.

I walked up to her.

"Give me a sec," she said, sensing I was there. "I'm basking in the moment."

Take some time to bask in who you are, what you've created, and how far you've come.

As our spiritual practice develops, we learn to separate from self, and to avoid attachment to any label Ego identifies with. We are more than a doctor or lawyer, more than a husband or parent. We exist beyond all of these labels. If your career were to end tomorrow, you would still be *you.*

However, as this part of our journey develops, we often forget to notice our life and to take a moment to bask in it. We're so busy working and creating, we rarely see the life we're living, and what we've created.

So take a look at your life from an outsider's perspective. Notice where you live and how you spend your time. See those choices you've made that helped you get to where you are. Notice how your home and clothing signify your choices. See your own paint-splotched overalls, and then spend some time basking in it. Dress it, see it, feel it. Don't just exist in it.

Claim your power. Recognize what you do. Realize how far you've come.

Take some time to bask in who you are, what you've created, and how far you've come.

Week Eighteen: **Start Small, and Stay Small if You Like**

My grandmother was magical. She could grow anything, from mighty trees to even mightier herb gardens. As a child, I would walk through the gate to her immense garden feeling like I had stepped into another world—one with wild blooms, heavenly scents, and, as every alternate world must have—a villain, which, in this case, were the bees.

As an adult, I tried many times to grow gardens equally ambitious as my grandmother's. But time and again, in my gardens, plants withered and died before harvest. So, I declared myself a black thumb, and thought it best to avoid growing any plants.

Until one day, quite by accident, I began growing daffodils in my worm farm. I had simply snuck the bulbs in for the winter, but through the care of my worms—heating pads on cold winter nights, mushroom soil, and non-chlorinated water—the bulbs sprouted. I watched in awe as the flowers grew, thriving under my care.

Two important lessons came from this. One was to start small. When I planted gardens nearly the size of my grandmother's, I was overwhelmed. They were simply too much work to upkeep.

But it was the next lesson that was even more important: Staying small is okay, too.

Who's to say that more brings more pleasure?

Three little bulbs in my worm farm brought me immense amounts of joy. But that doesn't mean more plants in a bigger garden will equal even more joy.

Start small, and stay small if it makes you happy. We don't always have to reach for more. Bigger is not always better.

Remember, we have nothing to prove to anyone or to ourselves. Don't deny yourself the joy in front of you because you think it isn't enough. If it brings you joy, it is exactly the right size.

So enjoy your flowerpot as my grandmother did her garden.

Week Nineteen: **The Key to Everything is Layers**

"The key to everything," the woman whispered to me as I passed by her on a busy street in the West Village, "is layers."

Although it was odd, I couldn't get her advice out of my mind. Later that night when I was back in my apartment, I thought about what she said, and I realized she was right. Layers are the key to so many things, from make-up application to conversations, cooking, flavors, writing, personalities, and life.

So why then, do we shun layers in our lives? Why do we limit ourselves, striving to be just one thing? It's as if we've branded ourselves as one particular type of person with one affiliation, and only one profession. And once we're aligned with this, we're unable to change.

But life is a vertical journey, not a horizontal one.

Every decision we make stands on the shoulders of the last. Inviting layers into our lives means creating an interesting, *holistic* life.

Week Twenty: **Build Your Internal Greenhouse**

An Internal Greenhouse is something you create inside of you to grow and nurture your dreams.

A greenhouse is a fixture that's built to create an optimal growing environment for plants, veggies, and flowers. In the greenhouse, the seeds have everything they need to sprout and flourish.

The same concept is true for your Internal Greenhouse. You need to create an environment inside of you that grows and nurtures your dreams.

Think of your dreams as seeds. You need to plant the seeds into a hospitable soil, water them, give them food, sunlight, and just like that, you've created ideal conditions for your seeds to become seedlings. From there, proper care will grow your seedling into a plant that flowers and offers you beauty or nourishment. Or both.

To chase your dreams, you need to be prepared physically and mentally. You need to create an environment where your intangibles can take root and thrive.

External circumstances will never be perfect. Phones will be ringing, kids screaming, dogs barking, coworkers texting, storms will roll in, and time will fly by. Despite all of those outside stressors, your Internal Greenhouse has to be as healthy as possible. Like the seeds, you need an environment to cultivate your dreams.

Just as the external circumstances will rarely be ideal, your Internal Greenhouse will also be challenged. That's where the work comes in. You'll have to fight for those things you need to sustain a healthy Internal Greenhouse—like: time, peace, relaxation, and, especially, joy.

Internal Greenhouse first appeared in How to Be Happier: 10 Action Steps You Can Use Every Day, also by Cathrine Goldstein

One day we wake up and realize that this is really all that there is. What we do in a day, the million little decisions we make, the birds we hear, the coffee we drink, the people we kiss goodnight.

Each thing that we do, each experience that we have, is as relevant as the rest.

Our journeys create our lives.

So, if we want to lead a life filled with love and happiness, then we must choose love and happiness in those million little decisions we make every single day.

When we choose to help someone else rather than ignoring them, we are choosing love. When we decide to forgive rather than staying angry, we are choosing love. And when we abandon worry, and embrace the simple act of being, we are choosing love.

And every time we choose love, our journey creates a life worth living.

Week Twenty-Two: **You Are Allowed to Change**

Change is a natural part of growth and life. You are changing at all times, but sometimes, the people closest to you, or even those you may not know at all, do not want you to change. They see it as a threat—after all, they have grown comfortable with the you they know, how dare you change?

Sometimes change is significant—maybe we've done something we're not proud of, and, vowing to never do that again, we've continued on in a different direction. Maybe we've left behind substances that were damaging our bodies, or work that was harming our souls.

Other times, change may not be noticeable to others, like the decision to pause and breathe.

Whatever change is coming for you, remember, you owe your life and life decisions to no one.

You are allowed to change:

Your mind

Your job

Your look

Your efforts

Your location

Your plan

Your life.

Your life is yours to be lived. Your life is not about making another feel any one way, or staying the way they imagine you. No matter what society tells you, you are not a brand. You are a person with this one life, and you owe it to no one to be any one way.

Your life is yours, and you are allowed to change.

Week Twenty-Three: **Rebrand Your Past**

The brilliant Nora Ephron once lamented that she had a million incredible experiences, but couldn't remember most of them.

From my perspective, this lack of remembering had nothing to do with aging or losing brain power. It had everything to do with a life crammed full of experiences, only some of which made it to memory.

We often remember the negative things that happen in our lives—we're biologically built that way. Survival of the species once relied on remembering and avoiding the "bad." And we're still wired that way today.

But we have a choice.

Many of us build our adult lives on "overcoming" challenges that happened to us in the past. But what if, instead of identifying with the bad, we looked between the lines and saw the good?

What if we "rebranded" ourselves to be the person who is entirely grateful for the many wonderful opportunities offered to us?

Consider your life as a whole. Remember your access to fresh air and healthy foods, to education, to a house and clothing, to relationships and employment. They probably weren't perfect, but that's exactly the point.

Now, make a conscious decision to be grateful for these things—not the lessons learned from the times you were hurt—just gratitude for life and the many opportunities

you've been given. No, the hurtful times won't magically
go away, but they don't have to define you.

*The simple act of gratitude can shift our perspective from
victim to victor, and rebranding ourselves can be as simple
as looking between the lines, and seeing the positive.*

Week Twenty-Four: **Be Kind**

Most of us have met with unkindness in our lives. At some point, there was someone who purposefully harmed us in some way.

Most of us can remember what that unkindness felt like. Maybe it still sits in our body, stored in our tissues and cells, and just remembering the harm can cause us distress. Most of us would never want to feel that way again.

So, be kind. Remember what it feels like to hurt and do not let that darkness into your soul ever again. If someone else hurts you, choose to let it go. Do not hurt them back. Being unkind to another life ultimately elicits the same negative result – it creates a world of pain and suffering.

Instead, rise above.

Be kind to kittens and puppies. To the elderly and children. Be kind to the driver who cut you off on the road and the person who cut you in line at the grocery store. Be kind to those who do not have the same values as you, and be kind to those who have hurt you—terribly. Be kind to all other life and lifeforms, be kind to Mother Earth, and, above all, be kind to yourself.

Dare to imagine a world where everyone is kind. That world starts with you.

Week Twenty-Five: **Only Light Can Drive Away Darkness**

"Darkness cannot drive out darkness; only light can do that. Hate cannot drive out hate, only love can do that."
– Martin Luther King, Jr.

What is that moment you are holding on to? That moment that's burned into your brain? What is that trauma that you relive time and again, whether you're alone walking through the woods, or lying in bed late at night?

What do you need to let go of? To forgive? Why is it so incredibly hard?

Despite my best efforts to let go and forgive, I carried my traumas with me everywhere. I imagined them crammed into an already overstuffed bag that was tied tight around my neck. The bag was so heavy that on some days, it prevented me from taking even a single step forward.

Then, one day, I realized that I was trying to drive out my darkness with more darkness. Although I was doing my best to forgive, *I was still sitting in the darkness of my past.*

Once I began to allow in the light, everything changed. Suddenly, instead of sitting in the dark, blindly groping for an explanation, I could let it go. I had stepped into the light. How? By doing something for someone else.

I may never understand why my traumas happened, but I can depower them by turning my focus away from them. Not by burying them, or denying them, but simply by doing something positive for someone else. Chances are, that someone else is battling traumas of their own as well.

Maybe, if we all came together and stepped into the light, if we truly cared for and helped one another, we could collectively see the good in the now, rather than blindly staring into the darkness of our past.

Only light can drive away darkness. Shine your light, and use it as a beacon to help others find their way.

Week Twenty-Six: **Love Like That**

I had never before seen a moment so beautiful captured by a picture.

A man celebrating his ninety-fifth birthday was hugging his daughter. His eyes were closed while a tear slid down his cheek, and his mouth was open to offer an escape for the overwhelming combination of the pain, and ecstasy, of love. The expression on his face was complete gratitude for life, joy of the moment, and love for his daughter.

It was love that made the deep grooves on his face seemingly fall away.

It was love that compelled him to hold her like that.

It was love that created such a bond.

I wish you love like that.

Love exists as so much more than simply romantic love. It exists in any way that you allow it.

I hope you are overcome by love. A love that gives itself freely and openly—that wears its heart not just on its sleeve, but on its whole being. I hope you find another to share the agony and bliss that coexist in any love story. I hope another holds you so tightly that you feel love, too.

I wish you love like that.

I wish you the freedom to love like that.

Week Twenty-Seven: **Your One Job is to Be Happy**

I sat across from an elderly woman on the subway who was smiling. The train was crowded, and people were glued to their phones, ignoring one another except for the occasional bump or push.

I couldn't stop looking at the smiling, older woman. She was dressed in a casual tweed suit and carried a small bag that she held on her lap—but it was the expression she wore that was captivating. She looked peaceful, content, and… happy. After a few stops the train emptied some, and glancing at me, the woman patted the empty plastic seat next to her.

Sitting next to her, I inhaled the scent of chicken soup and moth balls.

Then she turned to me. "We all have one job in this life," she told me. "That is, to be happy." Then she got up and left at the next stop, leaving me to wonder what she meant.

Through the years I have pondered those words, and now, I believe I finally understand what the woman was telling me.

Life is finite. If we spend our days miserable, we lose precious time. Life is not about work, or collecting items that may mean nothing to us in a month's time. It's not about leaving a mark on the world or rising to the top of anything.

The purpose of life is to be truly and deeply happy—maybe not at all moments, but overall. We were granted this astonishing gift of life, so why would we take it for granted? Our job is to appreciate it and enjoy it. Simply. That's all. Why would we choose to take this gift and spend it in any other way?

Your one job in this life is to be truly, deeply happy.

Week Twenty-Eight: **Let Your Home Smell**

Let your home smell of garlic and onions. Grow herbs in colorful pots and play jazz through opened windows. Let last week's tomato sauce dot your backsplash, as you hum, busily stirring this week's batch.

Stop worrying about keeping everything tidy, or it being neat and clean. *We spend too much of our lives worrying that we've become too much, when really, we've only just begun to tap into our true potential.*

So sing, dance, move the stack of books from your table to your counter. Forget to sweep, free yourself from the confines of being small. Of being proper.

Let your heart free and your soul will follow.

Week Twenty-Nine: **I Am Done With That**

Like you, I have spent a lot of time contemplating forgiveness. We understand that forgiving is essential for healing, and we know that to move on, we have to forgive. Forgiveness is about no longer carrying the weight of our pain, not about the one who has hurt us.

But sometimes, forgiving is too difficult a task. The word itself is charged with subtext and carries so much intention, that just the idea of forgiving, and all the work it entails, seems exhausting.

In those times, put down the idea of forgiveness, and instead, tell yourself: *I am done with that.*

I am done with that, allows you to walk away from the incident on your terms. It gives you your power back, and it gives you the power to make a break from the pain. This is your opportunity to be free.

When forgiveness is too great a concept to tackle, simply tell yourself, I am done with that. *Whatever that was, it's over now. Tell yourself,* I can choose to step away from it. I can choose to move on with my life. I am distancing myself and leaving it behind. It was a thing of my past, but I am done with that, and every step I take away from the pain, is a step toward my freedom.

Week Thirty: **You Do Not Need Permission**

Who told you that someone else had authority over you?
Did this idea stem from your parents or other adults when
you were young? Did it come from teachers who demanded
obedience in exchange for your education, or an entitled
boss who expected your gratitude in trade for your
paycheck? Or maybe it was general worry and anxiety that
taught you it was better to wait for permission than to trust
your own instincts…?

Who told you that you could be denied *anything* just
because they said so? Whether it be your freedom, your
education, or your livelihood?

Well it's not true. Any of it. In fact, the truth is:

*Once you become an adult, no one has control over you
except you.*

But autonomy walks hand in hand with bravery.

You don't need anyone's permission, but you do need to be
brave. Brave enough to listen to that voice inside that
knows best. The voice that knows when it's time to leave
your job, or fight for a relationship. The voice that tells you
when you need to keep going, and when you need to rest.

*That voice knows everything you need to know, all you
have to do is to trust.*

Week Thirty-One: **Control is Not a Bad Word**

In all of us, there exists an ongoing dance between creation and pause. Time when we move forward and time when we may choose to reflect. In those times of pause and reflection, we may see ourselves and our lives clearly. And we may not like what we see.

We may say, "The Universe brought me here. So I am meant to be here, right now." This is true. But it's also true that you had a hand in every decision you've made on the way.

Trust the Universe, but also trust that the Universe wants you to be happy. Trust that you have free will and have made choices. Although no choice is wrong (all experiences teach us something), there may be a particular experience that is no longer serving you.

So, if you feel like you're headed down the wrong path, change it.

If you feel like life is happening to you and you are not in control of your own life—*take back your control.*

Control is *not* a bad word. It's true that we have no control over circumstances or others. But we do have ultimate control over ourselves.

If you are headed down a path that does not serve you physically, mentally, emotionally, artistically, or spiritually, change it. The Universe will make sure you end up where you need to be, but the way you get there is completely under your control.

Week Thirty-Two: **Jealousy**

Jealousy is a complex emotion, and even though it gets a bad rap, it serves a purpose.

When we feel jealous toward someone else, toward something they have, or even more so, have accomplished, it's the Universe offering us a wake-up call.

It's a not-so-subtle cue—a road sign on our life's path—and it means we should pay attention.

We're not jealous of most things in life. We're not jealous of our neighbor's ski trip if we hate the cold, or our coworker's promotion when we were planning to leave the company anyway.

In fact, often we experience *Mudita*, the very opposite of jealousy. At those times, we're genuinely thrilled for a fellow human, simply because they've accomplished something great.

That's why, when we feel jealousy, we need to look at it, layer by layer.

What is it we are truly jealous of? Someone's success? Their happiness? Close your eyes and connect with your heart. What is it telling you? What is it you really want?

Jealousy is our own personal sherpa, guiding us toward the mountain and showing us the path. But once we've found our way, it's time to thank Jealousy, and let it go. What was meant for someone else was not meant for us in the exact same way.

When we experience jealousy and then let it go, we're left with knowledge we can use to better our lives. Maybe our jealously unearthed a desire we never knew we had, or a direction we didn't know our heart wanted to take.

Jealousy serves a purpose, to guide you and to let you know that you need to make a shift in your life—maybe even a change of course.

Week Thirty-Three: **It's Not You, It's Them**

"It's so nice to be around a woman who eats," one of my dinner companions said. He was speaking to another woman, one who was new to our group. As she blushed and began pushing food around her plate, he glanced at me. It was only for a second, but I knew what he was insinuating. What I chose to put into my body (or not into my body) was a cause of distress for him.

Why? Deep inside, my dinner companion must have been worried about his own food choices, and my choice to eat a plant-based, animal-free, alcohol-free diet upset him.

My choices caused an unsettled feeling in my dinner companion, one that was so uncomfortable, he chose to try to make two other people more uncomfortable than he was.

When someone makes a negative remark about you, understand it has nothing to do with you.

Your power lies in realizing that the problem they have is theirs. My vegetarian diet bothered my dinner companion because he felt bad about his own food choices. By calling out another woman, he not only embarrassed her, but tried to take *his* mind off of his guilt by causing strife at the table.

When someone insults you or compliments you in an offhanded way, understand this is not about you. Close your eyes, take a breath, and silently wish them well. What you choose to do with your life is for you—and only you—to decide.

You cannot change your path to please someone else. Know yourself, respect yourself. Make choices that are right for you and stay true to them. Another person is not yours to "fix." They have their journey, you have yours. So nod politely at your companion, and remind yourself, "It's not me. It's them."

Week Thirty-Four: **People Can Be Assholes** *

When we were filing paperwork to adopt our youngest child, we saw a Notary Public who purposely botched her signature on our paperwork. She smiled while she scribbled, laughed when she handed the paper to me, and smirked a "good luck." Her behavior set our adoption process back months.

I didn't know this woman, we had no personal history, and as far as I knew, there was no grudge she was holding against me. For years I wondered about this—I could not imagine why she would do something so very hurtful to all parties, especially our child. And then one day, in meditation, it came to me.

People can be assholes.

But, if every person in our life comes to us for a reason, what reason is there for assholes?

As I sat on my meditation cushion, I asked myself that very question. And I proceeded to ask that question for the next decade.

Finally, I received an answer:

Even assholes come into our lives for a reason, the thing is, we may never know why. And that's okay.

What a liberating realization that was.

We don't have to know why someone is in our life. We don't have to decipher every lesson that comes our way.

That's where the power of choice comes in. I will probably never know why that Notary purposefully tried to hinder our adoption process, but does it really matter?

The adoption went through, our daughter is home, and chances are, we will never see that woman again. So it's time to let it go. Asking why she did what she did only serves to hurt us.

Letting go of past wrongs can be difficult, but accepting that you don't need to know why they happened, can help.

People can be assholes (any of us, at any given time), but the trick is to accept that fact, and then, to simply let go.

Yoga Teachers: Feel free to substitute another word for "asshole." Any word that fits your class.

Week Thirty-Five: **Freedom Comes From Inside**

I sat there missing New York City in my very bones. I needed to get back—to the place I spent the majority of my life. It wasn't like the city was calling to me, it was like *I was calling to it* from my soul. Monotony had created an inner vibration deep inside of me, and although all I craved was freedom, I could not free myself. I needed help—I needed to be dropped into the heart of the city I loved and allowed to ride the wave of each and every heartbeat.

So, I decided I would drag my family with me despite their objections. Just for a weekend, just for a break. As I sat there googling things for teens in NYC, an ad popped up in the corner of my screen—it was to visit a farm somewhere, far from NYC, where you could swim with pigs.

My soul perked up. "That's it!" it screamed. "That's where we need to go!" A farm. The polar opposite of New York City.

And suddenly, I realized… I did not really need New York City, or a farm in the middle of nowhere. I needed to go inward, and to find out why I felt so very trapped.

The most important journey is the journey we take inward. Travel is good for the soul, but it's only a temporary escape. If you're feeling caught, or trapped, the only answer is to turn inward and find out why. No amount of distraction can "cure" you of this feeling.

True freedom can only come from inside.

Week Thirty-Six: **You Can't Contain Spirit**

Your spirit is you and you are your spirit. Your spirit cannot be stopped or contained, and for as long as you are alive, it can't be altered or exterminated.

But, our spirits can be seen as dangerous entities by those in our lives. Sometimes, we see spirit in someone we love and grow angry. We know that spirit will take them away from us and the safety of the home we've created for them, and we panic.

"How can this be?" we ask. "I've created a world for you—a home in the safest neighborhood, a relationship where your needs are met. Why are you leaving?"

But in these moments we need to consider that we may have created this world for *us*, and not really for them. In this beautiful prison we've built for them, we can worry less.

The truth is, no matter how tightly we hold on, the one thing we cannot contain is spirit. Not theirs, and not ours, either.

Our children will leave the safety of their home, our partners and families will follow the call of their spirits. They have to, it is the only way they can live.

And what of us?

Your spirit is no different. Maybe your spirit has been ignored for some time, but it's still there, bubbling and waiting in anticipation. It wants nothing more than to lead you to your life's calling.

Sit quietly. Close your eyes. Turn inward. That inner voice you hear is your guide. Listen to it as carefully and earnestly as you would a guide as you ascend Mt. Everest, because nothing is more important than this.

Your spirit cannot be contained.

Support and applaud others as they follow their spirits, and listen to yours. Your spirit will always break free of its confines, and lead you exactly where you need to go.

Week Thirty-Seven: **Be Inspired**

To manifest our dreams, we have to stay inspired. Sometimes, it can be a lot to create our own magic. Luckily, the world is made to be an endless source of inspiration.

Inspiration can come at any time and from any place, but we have to be open and receptive. Sometimes, following all the golden rules: breathwork, meditation, sitting quietly and listening, isn't enough. We're just too exhausted to rely completely on ourselves for inspiration. Sometimes, we need to turn outward, not inward.

There's no shame in needing to turn outward for inspiration. The world was designed as a playground for our senses, after all. For centuries, great artists have learned from other great artists.

So take yourself out. Listen to the birds. The raging river, the music of a local band. Go to a crowded city or an empty field.

It doesn't matter what it is, but take yourself out and let yourself be inspired.

Week Thirty-Eight: **Simplify Your Life**

No matter what age you are or what you've accomplished, no matter what time of the year it is, there's a good chance you are ready to simplify your life.

How do you simplify?

First, take a moment to consider: where is my life overly complicated? Where have I spread myself too thin? Where am I burning the candle at both ends?

Then ask yourself, what would simplifying my life mean to me?

There are no right answers, and no rules to simplifying your life, but there is an important distinction:

Simplifying is not a synonym for minimalism, or for decluttering.

In our society, the concepts of minimalism and decluttering often come with so many rules they can stress us out—leaving us with the exact opposite result of what we wanted.

Truthfully, sometimes we don't need to clear something from our lives. Sometimes, to simplify our lives, we need to add something—support, help, a community, or even an item that can help us to live an easier, fuller life.

Simplifying your life is different for every person, but it always comes down to one thing: how can this act of simplifying—whether it's clearing or adding—better serve you...?

Week Thirty-Nine: **Live in Your Life of Now, Not Someday**

I was walking through the downstairs of my house making a mental checklist of what needed to be cleaned or tossed, what I could rearrange, and how I would redecorate.

My mind and body were distanced from one another as I planned for what my house would look like Someday. Someday, I would hang Deruta pottery on my already cluttered kitchen walls. Someday, I would replace the chairs. Someday, I would really live here.

Then it hit me. There is no someday. There is only now.

I had been existing in my house—a house where I was raising my children—without *really living in it* at all.

And, if this was true of the way I lived in my house, was it true of the way I lived my life as well?

How many of us exist without really living?

The time to start living is now. Immediately. There will never be a moment when everything is right. The walls may be cluttered and the chairs old, but they are a part of life. Exactly as life is meant to be, right now.

Make peace with your life as it is. Greet it like the stranger it may be, but embrace it like the old friend it truly is. Stop worrying, planning, and distancing. Above all, change "when" into "now," and *live* in your life.

Week Forty: **Don't Forget to Live Today**

One of my most profound spiritual lessons came when I was nineteen years old and working in a biker bar in Hell's Kitchen, New York City. The bar employed a bunch of theatre kids who didn't want to be there (me, included), and one really grumpy manager. When any of the theatre kids would announce an upcoming audition or play reading, the manager would remind us that we were not, in fact, actors or playwrights—we were really "only" cocktail waitresses and bartenders.

Although the manager meant what he said in the most unsupportive of ways, his message actually contained an important lesson in yoga and in life:

When we live only in the future, we forget to live in the present, and we miss out on life.

Living in the present does not mean we don't plan and dream. But when we hold our breath and wait for that next thing that will save us from our current situation—we set ourselves up for disappointment. There is no job or success that can offer us salvation. We are not one step away from happiness. Our salvation lives inside of us. Our happiness is within us.

So plan for the future, but don't forget to live today.

Week Forty-One: **You are Your Own CEO**

If you worked for a company that had a CEO, you'd
probably listen to what that person had to say about the day
to day running of the company. Chances are, that person
had either started the company, or they were brought on
because of their expertise in the field. And, to remain as an
effective CEO, that person would have to listen to the
heartbeat of the company, honor its truth, and follow its
mission statement, all while supporting it through growth
and change.

It's no different for you. *You are your own CEO.*

Imagine you are a company with different departments:
body, mind, and spirit. You also have a personalized
mission statement—your overall goal, your life's purpose,
or dharma.

As you grow and age, changes naturally take place in your
company. In addition, your company will hopefully expand
as you find many different ways to live in your dharma.

Since we have the most intimate knowledge of ourselves,
why do we listen to everyone—and anyone—before we
listen to ourselves? Why is it difficult to trust ourselves?
Because we're conditioned to believe everyone knows
better than us, even when it comes to a topic we know
best—ourselves.

We know the truth about ourselves. We know what's right
for us and what isn't, but when we stop trusting, we go off
track.

Listen to yourself. Trust yourself. No one knows you or what's right for you, better than you do.

You are your own CEO.

Week Forty-Two: **Don't Try So Hard**

If you've ever forgotten something—the name of an actor
in that movie you once loved, or a point you were trying to
make—then you know forcing yourself to remember
doesn't work. When you push to remember something
you've forgotten, you send signals to your body to tense—
maybe you squeeze your eyes shut or ball your fists. Then
your mind begins to focus on the fact that you've forgotten,
rather than on *what* you've forgotten. Once that starts,
panic sets in, and the elusive answer slides even farther
away.

Suddenly, hours later, while you're shampooing your hair
or driving down the street, the answer pops into your head.
Not only the answer, but the greatest idea for a book
anyone has ever had. *In the history of the world.*

Why did inspiration decide to strike now? While your
hands are occupied with other things? Because you've
given up the struggle. You've relaxed and breathed. And
you've stopped trying so hard.

Creation needs freedom and space. We can no more force
ourselves to create than we can to remember. The
inspiration we seek while creating can be as elusive as the
long-lost thought. We cannot force an answer.

Creativity comes when we relax and breathe. When we
allow room for our inner voice to speak, and for Source to
deliver inspiration.

*The next time you need to remember something or are
feeling caught; the next time you are desperate for
inspiration—stop. Take a deep breath, a long walk, or a*

yoga class. Allow your body and mind the freedom to answer.

Week Forty-Three: **The Times of Darkness Are There to Show Us the Light**

Sometimes the darkness feels like a weighted blanket covering us from crown to toe. It's heavier and denser than the thickest fog, and as we crawl farther under our blanket, we can't imagine there will ever be a way out. And sometimes, we are so tired and so disheartened, we don't want one.

But those times of darkness are there to show us the light.

Darkness is one way our soul communicates with us.

Darkness is there to show us that what we are doing isn't right for us. That our long beaten path needs a change. Darkness serves as a giant neon highlighter scribbling over the manuscript of our lives announcing "Pay attention!" and "This isn't okay!"

Those times of darkness are there to show us the light.

To show us that our hearts are unhappy. That our souls want more. Learn to embrace the darkness as a time to be quiet and still. Just listen. There is so much more for you than what you see. There is so much more meant for you than what you're doing. No matter what your age, you haven't yet truly begun to live your life. You're only now starting to understand your purpose by feeling what isn't right for you.

Those times of darkness are there to show us the light.

Although they are difficult, honor the times of darkness and your feelings about them. Learn from the darkness. It is there to show you the light.

Week Forty-Four: **Being Blocked is a Gift**

Throughout my career, I have worked with many writers who have been "blocked." These writers have something they want to write, or need to write, but the words simply will not come. In response, I have led meditations, yoga classes, breathwork, chakra-balancing, and one-on-one sessions, all to help them free their blockages.

What I've come to realize is that I was wrong in trying to release these mental blocks, because blocks are a gift.

Blocks are there for a reason.

Whether you are an artist, a businessperson, a student, or are on a journey to find yourself, think of a time you've been blocked. We all experience it. It's a horrible feeling—maybe you believed you were unable to do that next thing, or dreaded the work you had to do, or maybe you felt whatever you were doing just wasn't "right."

Now, consider the work that block surrounded. Chances are, it was something that went against your core beliefs. No, it may not have been a direct line to one of your truths, but it probably touched on it in some way.

Now when I work with a writer who is blocked, I ask them, "Why? What is it about this particular book or post that you do not align with?" Sometimes the answer is clear, and sometimes the answer is hidden behind a lack of inspiration. But that very lack of inspiration is a clue that you are not living in a way that is true for you.

So, the next time you feel blocked in life, ask yourself, "Why? What is it about this particular responsibility that goes against my fundamental beliefs?" Or, "Is this job simply wrong for me at this time in my life? Why?"

Then turn inward and listen to the answer. In that answer lies a cue to your soul.

The next time you are feeling blocked, remember, being blocked is a gift.

Every block can be the messenger of what your soul wants you to know.

Week Forty-Five: **They Meant to Hurt You, AND It Doesn't Matter**

People hurt us. They call us names, or inflict physical harm. They purposefully sabotage us at work, or leave us when we're counting on them the most.

In response, we're told that no one can really hurt us; it's our choice how we allow ourselves to be affected by someone. We're told that to put the hurt behind us, we have to forgive people and maybe even empathize. Hurt people, hurt people, after all. Chances are, they never meant to hurt us to begin with.

But that's not realistic, and may not be entirely truthful.

The truth is, they may have meant to hurt you, AND it doesn't matter.

You alone have the power to recognize this and step away from the pain. Yes, they may have meant to hurt you. Yes, you may have been hurt. Yes, it was ultimately your choice to be hurt (you could have chosen not to be), and yes, they may have known hurt in their past, and that was their reason for hurting you.

Still, none of it matters. All that matters is that you move on. Pain in our past is to be left in our past, otherwise, we replay this pain over and over, and begin to become inseparable from it. I am my pain, and my pain is me.

To move on, we have to let go. There's no need to dress up our pain in silk robes and feather boas, or to scrutinize it in the middle of a sacred circle on a moonlit night.

Instead, simply open your hand and allow the pain to float away. If you're ready to say goodbye, then say goodbye. Because, *they may have meant to hurt you, AND it really doesn't matter to you at all.*

Week Forty-Six: **Self-Care is Not One Size Fits All**

For the longest time I thought I was broken.

When everyone else ran to the quiet woods or beach for self-care, my soul craved the noise of the city. One look down at the streets decorated with litter, followed by one quick glance up at the lights so bright they blocked out the stars, and I could finally relax.

The city calmed me, but time and time again, I was taught that it shouldn't. Self-care meant escaping for a walk in the woods, or being alone under the night sky. Never did any self-help guru announce, "You should recharge in the hustle and bustle of a city." Deciding there was something wrong with me, I tried to conform.

Then one day, as stress enveloped me like an unrelenting tsunami, I began driving and didn't stop until I found myself in the middle of a city. Turning off the car, I felt myself relax—my heart had finally found peace.

Self-care is care for your *self*.

Self-care does not mean following the latest trend. By its very definition, it should mean something different for each of us.

Forget what you've been told. Instead, ask yourself: What calms my heart when I'm feeling stressed? What ignites my passion when I'm feeling stuck? What can I do right now that will make me happy?

This is how we truly begin to practice self-care.

Week Forty-Seven: **Go Where Your Soul Leads You**

Imagine, just for a moment, that social media was gone. Imagine that nothing you did or said had to be recorded or put on display for likes and comments. Imagine that all that was required of you was to live—and I mean *truly live*—your life without the approval of anyone.

What would you do? Where would you go? How would your life be different?

There is a quiet pull that begins in your heart, and calls you forth. Those pictures of cornfields you can't stop staring at, the hiking trail you're itching to walk, the trip to India that won't leave your mind…this is where your soul beckons to go.

This place your soul tells you about, it is only a stop along your journey, not your final destination. But still, in this place, you'll uncover your truest self.

This pull is the calling of your soul. Listen to it.

Go to where your soul leads you, and you will never be wrong.

Week Forty-Eight: **You're All My Favorites**

When my girls were little, my husband and I would read them a book about a mother and father bear who assured their baby cubs that there was no one favorite, rather, all of them were their favorites.

"But, how could we both be your favorite?" our girls asked. "There can only be one favorite."

We explained that we loved all parts of them and in all ways. As they were different people, they had different personalities, and we loved all parts of those personalities. None more than another. So, they were all our favorites.

Wouldn't it be wonderful to extend this same courtesy to ourselves and love all parts of ourselves equally?

The truth is, there are no good or bad parts of you. Yes, there are some parts you may only share with those you love most, but it's all of those parts together that make you, well, *you.*

So close your eyes, turn inside, and think of those things about yourself that you have learned to love less. Maybe you were told that you were selfish, lazy, or dishonest; called a liar or a fraud. Whatever they are, call those parts of you forward without judgment. Remember, all of these parts exist in all of us.

Now, take a deep breath and say, I accept you.

All parts of us make us who we are. Let go of favoritism within yourself.

Let your body, mind, and spirit know – you're all my favorites.

Week Forty-Nine: **You Do Know What to Do**

Every time you say to yourself, *I don't know what to do,* pause and listen.

You do know what to do.

Every time you doubt you have the answer. Pay attention.

It's there, in the deepest parts of you.

Every time you wonder which way to turn, or how you'll get by, trust.

You'll figure it out. You always do.

Have you always chosen the right path? Yes. It may not have been the easiest path, but it was the right one because it brought you to here, to this very moment.

Whenever you doubt, trust instead.

You do know what to do.

Week Fifty: **Be You, It's Enough**

Have you ever noticed that when we see a memory of someone missing their mother, they miss the woman who danced with them in the kitchen? Who calmed them down before a test or fought monsters in the closet?

Have you noticed when we see them missing their dad, we watch the memory of playing catch or making grilled cheese?

What we don't see is the moment Mom or Dad won an Academy Award or a Nobel Prize.

Take a moment and ask yourself, whom or what do you miss and why? Chances are, whomever and whatever you miss has to do with the little things. The real things. The intimacy between two living beings. The love that is shared.

The people who rely on you the most simply need you to be there for them. Not to be *something* for them. They just need you to be *you*.

This is true in all aspects of your life—including how you think of yourself. Achieving goals is wonderful, but understand that it doesn't make you more special.

Show up for others and yourself. Be kind, live your life fully and joyfully, and above all, be you, it's enough.

Week Fifty-One: **Sometimes It's Enough**

Sometimes it's enough to sit in the early sun on a cold winter morning and listen to the birds. Sometimes it's enough to marvel at the budding sky, the squirrels rushing back and forth, and the way the light filters through the branches of the tallest trees. Sometimes it's enough to hold your hands around a mug of steaming hot tea, and to watch as Mother Earth wakes, wrapping her arms around another day.

Sometimes it's enough to just be.

Week Fifty-Two: **Remember, There is Still So Much Good in the World**

On a particularly cold winter evening, we were delivering a carful of hot meals and warm coats to a men's homeless shelter at the end of a long, dead-end street. As we turned down the street, we spotted a group of tents and cardboard boxes—a makeshift camp located a short distance from the shelter.

We stopped to offer meals and coats, and a very large man with graying hair and a booming voice came directly to the car. He thanked us for what we were offering, and as he slipped into one of the coats, he explained that the shelter was full, and they were on the street for the night. The warm coats, blankets, and hot food were greatly appreciated.

A few minutes passed, and as we continued to speak, a much younger man—maybe still a boy—walked out of the camp and over to the car. Unfortunately, we had run out of coats and blankets, so we offered him a hot meal, which was all we had left.

"Thanks," he muttered, "it's really, really cold."

"It is," the older man agreed. Then he slipped out of his warm coat. "Here," he smiled at the young man and handed him the coat. "You're scrawny. It'll fit you better anyway."

The young man nodded as he pulled on the coat. Then the older man thanked us and disappeared into the camp.

Yes, the world is filled with war and violence. But there is still so much good. Even more, there is the *potential* for so much good in each of us. Whenever you doubt this, remember:

On the coldest of nights, one homeless man gave another homeless man the coat off of his back.

(Bonus) Week Fifty-Three: **You Are Here For a Reason**

If you've ever doubted that there was a reason you were born, talk to a friend who is having trouble conceiving. I was that friend who drank Chinese teas and went to acupuncture in no-name bodegas, who underwent operations, hormones, retrievals, multiple daily shots, over-stimulations, countless IUIs, three failed IVFs, and years of devastating heartbreak, all in the hopes of becoming pregnant and having children.

Ask that friend how difficult becoming pregnant can be.

Human life is an absolute miracle. The chances of one particular sperm and egg meeting at just the right time—something that even science cannot manipulate to guarantee a positive outcome—is awe-inspiring. Creating life takes a miracle. Your life took a miracle.

You are here for a reason.

Even on your darkest days—on days when it feels like all is lost. Even when it seems that the whole world is succeeding and you are not, remember:

You are here for a reason.

During those times when you feel caught in the monotony of life, and you can't see a way out, remember:

You are here for a reason.

Chances are, you don't know what that reason is. You may not see it. It may show itself to you in a day or a year, or maybe, never. But you are here for a reason. Trust that.

After all, you know what a miracle it was for you to be born.

Close your eyes and breathe it in.

You are here for a reason.

And that reason is big and bright and beautiful and powerful. The reason is global, and lifechanging. The reason is impactful.

Trust it.

You are here for a reason.

Poems

Privileged Enough for Poison

Her forehead is not privileged enough for poison.
Her hair isn't wealthy enough to change.
Her nails are not advantaged enough to shine.
Her face is too poor to turn unnaturally upward.
Her skin isn't favored enough to flatten…

But her soul!
Her mind!
Her dreams!
Her *understanding*.

Her journey.
Her faith.
Her belief.
Her courage.
Her fierceness.
Her trust.
Her determination.

Her glow.

Damn. Her *glow*.

Here's What I Know that I Wish You Knew

Here's what I know that I wish you knew:
Your ass is your ass whether it's covered in hundreds of
dollars or dozens of dollars
Nails aren't meant to be any one color
It's okay if hair moves
Food isn't really the devil

You're perfect exactly as you are.

A Beautiful Soul

If she were a map,
she'd be filled with mountains and valleys
roadwork, and unknown final destinations

For years I followed this beautiful soul
wondering what made her so dynamic
now I see.
She is her.
Truthfully
and honestly
and messily
and beautifully

Change

Embrace the changes the Universe sends your way
even, and especially, when they seem finite and painful
those are the easy ones
the ones where we feel we have
no responsibility in decision making
those changes – no matter what – are a gift

I'm Not Here

I'm not here for you to fix
or change
I'm not here to be pulled from the abyss by cheerleaders
wielding self-help books
and I don't want your pep talk.

It's okay that I'm here
It's okay I'm not fixed
It's okay that I don't know what's next

It's okay.
I'm okay.
Exactly as I am.

Who You Want Me to Be

I spent a lifetime being who you wanted me to be. I tried to be smarter, dumber, taller, and shorter, but I couldn't keep it going. I fought as hard as I could to stay, and swam against the raging currents. I changed and adapted to your every whim, but I never succeeded. Then one day, you were gone, and I was no one, I thought.

Until, finally, I became me.

For Once and For All

For once and for all,
stop judging yourself.

You're not too loud
or too bossy.
You're not too big
or too small.

You're not stupid
or mean

Yes, sometimes
you're forgetful, late, careless
and sometimes, you're even all of these at once.
Sometimes you hurt someone without knowing it,
or say the wrong thing,
and sometimes you react without thinking.

But…

You're neither hopeless
nor reckless
You didn't Mess up
Screw Up
or F—up.

You simply did.
The best you could and the best you can.

And doing *is* what matters.

For once and for all, stop judging you.

Someday

"Someday," she decided, "I will yank off this weight hanging around my neck, and I will run free across the meadow. Someday, I will pull this heaviness off of my back, and do cartwheels through the daisies. Someday, I will be rid of this damned anchor that makes my shoulders slump and my chest cave in on itself. Someday, I will climb the tallest mountain, with no fear—or better yet, *plenty* of heart-pumping, adrenaline-coursing fear, but no *worry*. I will pull myself up by strong arms, throwing elbow after elbow, shimmying higher up the ice—body pressed tight against the cold, wet slickness, while I smile broader and brighter than I ever thought possible. Someday, I will seek out the highest peak and climb higher still. Someday, when I am at the very pinnacle of the mountain, I will pound my fists against my chest and howl at the golden moon. Someday, I will rid myself of these damned limitations of my youth, and I will finally yell, 'Enough!'"

"Someday," she decided, "is now."

New Home

When she was ready to move into her new home,
the first thing she unpacked was from her childhood.
It was that boy who called her a name because she didn't
look like him.
Or dress like him.
Because her mother worked the register at the Five and
Dime as they called it back then
and her father worked on other people's cars.
She took that boy out of the invisible suitcase she carried
on her back, shook him off, and let him go.

The next thing she unpacked was from her teen years.
She reached into her bag and with a gentle tug,
pulled forth the memory of the girls who said she couldn't
sit with them at lunch.
That she belonged somewhere else—anywhere else.
She held those girls up and stared at them long and hard,
and with a whisper of forgiveness,
she let them go.

Feeling lighter now and so much stronger,
she then unpacked her college boyfriend who had broken
her heart,
her first boss who yelled at her for sport, she was sure,
the series of dates that ended terribly
the jobs she abandoned
the man she was with when she should have known better,
the men she was with when she should have known better.

From her suitcase she yanked the memory of the extra
money she stole from the tip jar,
and the times she said she would be there and wasn't—

She freed all the "Wrong" things she said and did
and all the "Wrong" things that were done to her.

She held up
the memory of her father's death
and her mother's illness.
Each was wrapped in an extra thick protective layer of
guilt.
Pulling at the packaging, they unraveled quickly, so she let
them go, too.

Then, she placed each memory carefully on a quilt laid out
on the floor before her
and with one deep breath, she took them all in—the sorrow,
the guilt, the embarrassment, the shame, the solitude, the
pain—so, so much pain—and then, she breathed them out.

She did this again and again until the people and the jobs
and the memories were nothing more than dust in the palm
of her hand.

With one soft blow, they were all released,
and with a full heart and a free mind, she was home.

Life Lessons from a Semi-Old Broad

Say yes to:
1) Cake—of all types
2) Love—of all types

Say no to:
1) Anything you want to.

Surrender

I'd never given up
Surrender was not a word
I knew
Stronger than most
I stood tall when others did not
Falling
with eyes closed

That's how I survived.
Shutting down.

Then, when I had buried it all so deep that
the only place left to go was up
I turned my face upward
to the light
to the closest tree.

A tiny seed fell straight into my heart
the seed of life
the seed of truth
the seed of regeneration.

And suddenly I didn't see myself
with these people
nor apart.

Now I stand tall in a different way
and my surrender means something different

For now I surrender to the truth
that grows within my heart.

Don't Wait

My parents were Timidity and Fear

Timidity convinced me to hold back
to stay put
no matter what

Fear warned
you're safer here
but I wasn't

Because the greatest consequence
was to my soul

I should have gone
I should have tried
I should have lived

Maybe I should do better for you
then to tell you to embrace life with
Passion and Bravery.
But it's truly all I have.
Let them be your parents
even when you've grown too old
for need of me.

Listen to them.
Always.

There Comes a Time

There comes a time
when we no longer look left or right
we surely don't look back
only forward
ever forward
always forward
chasing what's been ours
all along.

The Wolf

The wolf dropped his head
and could no longer howl
at even the brightest
Hunter's Moon
on the coldest October night

Because surely the worst had happened

And yet, he limped home
and hunted for his food
and after eating to his fullest
he lay down to rest
as the moon set
on what was to become
bright day
once again

And once again,
the wolf stirred

My Path

My path isn't
long and picturesque,
it isn't made of cobblestones
and lined with
colorful leaves
that crunch
under my feet
leading me to the house
of answers

No matter how much
I may want it to be

My path is an LA freeway
filled with noise
and pollution
loops and turns

My path converges at places
it shouldn't
making traffic jams
that last not hours but
days

My path is filled with
potholes and closures
sometimes with road rage
and dead ends

My path is a tangled
mess of tries and misses

But still
it is my path

And it leads me
exactly
where I need to go

Be Strong, My Friend

Their words are like the strongest winds now
howling in your ear
shaking your very core

maybe they rip away
your shutters
that were once
blocking your view of the world
keeping you falsely safe

And yes, those wind-words hurt
no matter what they say

But nothing that ferocious
can last
except your spirit

Which, rising up like the
Great Goddess she is
holds her hands wide
until the wind-words
retreat into little
puffs of air
that may not be forgotten
but are gone.

Yes, by god. They are gone.

And you are here. And you are here.

All the Women that I Am

I want the chance to be all the women that I am.
With long, black hair and wild eyes;
to pray so hard for someone I love
my chest caves inward to hold my heart.

Every Moment

Suddenly, as I approached that mark of half a century, I understood. I was thankful for every moment I'd had— from my tortured youth, to my most blissful days brimming with chocolate and baby kisses.

I understood every moment was created just for me, so that I may have this one true voice, and I may share it with the world.

So now I am thankful for it all.

It didn't just make me who I am, but rather, who I am was the reason for it all.

And its sweetness and bitterness and clarity and vagueness, all of it was given to me so I may give back.

An Army of One

The truth is,
I ran
but the running brought me nowhere
except to where I was afraid
scared of who I was
scared that I didn't belong
that I didn't fit
that they'd hate me

But finally, I stopped running
and I listened to the stillness
and the quiet
and I stopped being afraid of the
sounds in my head
and I stopped being afraid of me

and in that moment
I knew I didn't have to run
I had to stay still
and go inward
to find peace there,
not in change
but in acceptance
and if they never do
find this acceptance of me
that's okay
Because I accept me
and I am an army of one
and that's all I've ever needed

So bow down, bullies
leave me, voices

taking fear and worry
with you
I am not running anymore
for now I understand

I am an Army of One

When I Wasn't Allowed to Live

When I wasn't allowed to live
Life was easier, somehow
Push back the tears that
weren't there
Stand tall against a wind
I didn't feel
Never Caring
Never Knowing

But now that I'm finally alive
Life is so much more
Devastating
And brilliant
And colorful
And passionate
And awe-inspiring

Now that I'm allowed to live
I never want to stop

Success

No one cared about
what I said
except me
No one liked
what I said
except me
No one gave praise
or stars
or recommendations
or promotions
or bought
or followed
except Me.

And it won't ever matter
to anyone
except me.

But it *does* matter. To me.

Me

Today I sat with the me of then and of next
I filled with warm light and wept for both.

I cried sadly for all the me of then had yet to experience.

     The sadness. The pain. The suffering.

When she looked at me, pink cheeks and giant eyes, I had
no answers.

How could I tell her what she still must face?

Then I saw the me of next. Old, wrinkled, small. I had that
certain smell that only age can bring.

She turned to the me of then and I cried for the joy she had
seen.

     And all that was to come.

I watched.
For only the me of next could assure the me of then.

And when she smiled, we two smiled with her.

This Time Upon the Earth

This time upon the earth is so short
I won't use it worrying about punctuation marks
Or getting it right
Or pants that no longer fit
Or making you happy

With my short time on this earth
I will say what I need to say
What I have to say
I will listen to the songs of the birds
And play too many games of *Uno*
I will hug the trees
And save the worms

It may not be pretty
I may not be pretty

Maybe it will affect you
Maybe not

And that's okay

Because my time upon this earth is
My time.

One last thing…

Don't forget to climb a mountain

and howl at the moon.

About the Author...

Cathrine Goldstein is a speaker and bestselling, award-winning author, playwright, and poet. A member of the International Association of Professional Wellness Coaches, she's a Holistic Wellness Coach and Dharma Coach, who practices her own brand of "Practical Wellness." She loves helping people chase their dreams, and she specializes in working with those who are looking to start over in their lives. A wife, mom, vegetarian, worm-farmer, and tree-hugger, she's also a long-time yoga instructor and studio manager. Cathrine has a Master's Degree in Theatre History, and is a proud member of the Dramatists Guild.

To work with Cathrine or for more information, please visit: MyDharmicJourney.com and @mydharmicjourney.

Books by Cathrine Goldstein...

Wellness/Poetry

When Dreams Become Memories, a Chapbook of Poetry

How to Be Happier: 10 Action Steps You Can Use Every Day (Available only at MyDharmicJourney.com)

Fiction/Young Adult

Cathrine is the author of numerous fiction and Young Adult novels, including *The Letting* series, as well as *The New York Artists* series, and *The New York Artists Series—After Dark*. She is also a ghostwriter of many novels.

You can find more information at: CathrineGoldstein.com

www.ingramcontent.com/pod-product-compliance
Lightning Source LLC
Chambersburg PA
CBHW072249260726
48659CB00004BA/1504